REVERSING CHRONIC KIDNEY DISEASE

A Simple Method On How To Avoid Dialysis and Improve Kidney Function

Dr Ruth T Todd

All Rights Reserved

The information in this book is for educational purposes only and is not intended to be a substitute for your physician. So therefore No part of this work may be reproduced, distributed, or transmitted in any form or by any means, including photocopying, recording, or other electronic or mechanical methods, without the prior written permission of the copyright owner, except in the case of brief quotations embodied in critical reviews and certain other noncommercial uses permitted by copyright law. Unauthorised reproduction, distribution, or use of this work may result in severe civil and criminal penalties, and will be prosecuted to the fullest extent permitted by law.

Copyright © Dr Ruth T. Todd 2023.

TABLE OF CONTENTS

Introduction..5
What Are Kidneys?... 9
    What is kidney disease?...................................9
    How is kidney disease diagnosed?...................... 10
    Stages of kidney disease?..................................11
    Symptoms of kidney disease?.............................15
    Causes of kidney disease............................... 16
Treatment for kidney disease..............................19
    Medications...20
    Diet.. 23
    Exercise...25
    Dialysis.. 27
    Kidney transplant...29
Prevention Of Kidney Disease............................ 33
Conclusion.. 35
    The future of kidney disease..............................35
    Hope and healing for people with kidney disease... 38

4

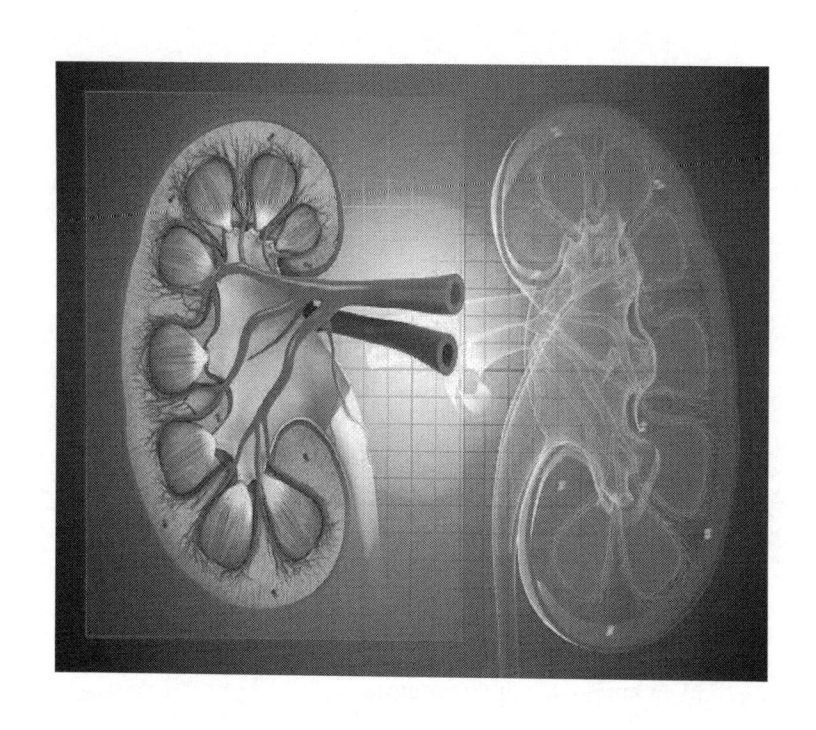

Introduction

The Reversing Kidney Disease is a book that provides a comprehensive guide to prevention, treatment, and recovery from kidney disease.

"The Kidney Disease Solution" is an essential resource for anyone who has kidney disease or who is at risk for developing kidney disease. The book provides clear and concise information on all aspects of kidney disease, and it offers practical advice on how to manage the condition.

If you have kidney disease, or if you are concerned about your risk for developing kidney disease, I highly recommend reading "The Kidney Disease Solution." This book can help you take control of your health and live a long and healthy life.

The Kidney Disease Solution covers a wide range of topics related to kidney disease, including:

* The causes of kidney disease
* The symptoms of kidney disease
* The stages of kidney disease
* The diagnosis of kidney disease
* The treatment of kidney disease
* The prevention of kidney disease

The book also includes a number of resources for people with kidney disease, including:

* A meal plan
* A yoga routine
* A meditation guide
* A symptom tracker

The reversing chronic Kidney Disease Solution is a valuable resource for people with kidney disease and their loved ones. The book provides information and guidance on how to manage kidney disease and live a healthy life.

The following are some of the book's most important lessons:

* Kidney disease is a serious condition, but it can be managed with proper treatment and care.

* If you have kidney disease, it is important to work with your doctor to create a treatment plan that is right for you.

* With proper care, you can live a long and healthy life with kidney disease.

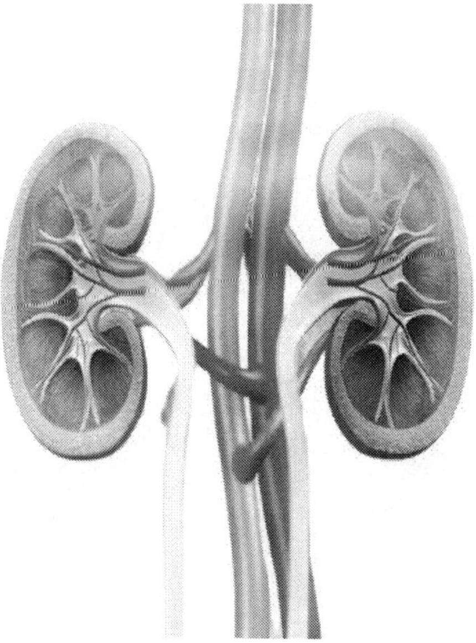

What Are Kidneys?

Kidneys are two bean-shaped organs that are located in the lower back, one on each side of the spine. They are in charge of generating urine and filtering waste materials from the blood. Kidneys also help to regulate blood pressure, blood sugar, and the body's fluid balance.

What is kidney disease?

Kidney disease is a condition that affects the kidneys and their ability to filter waste products from the blood. Kidney disease can be caused by a number of factors, including diabetes, high blood pressure, and chronic infections. If left untreated, kidney disease can lead to kidney failure, which is a life-threatening condition

How is kidney disease diagnosed?

Kidney disease is diagnosed with a combination of tests, including:

- **Blood tests:** Blood tests help to measure the amounts of waste products like urea and creatinine in the blood. One can use these values to gauge how well the kidneys are working.
- **Urine tests:** Urine tests can be used to check for protein in the urine, which can be a sign of kidney damage.
- **Imaging tests:** Imaging tests, such as an ultrasound or a CT scan, can be used to look at the kidneys and see if there are any signs of damage.
- **Kidney biopsy:** During a kidney biopsy, a small sample of kidney tissue is taken and seen under a microscope. This can be used to

diagnose kidney disease and determine the cause of the damage.

If you have any of the risk factors for kidney disease, or if you are experiencing any of the symptoms of kidney disease, it is important to talk to your doctor. Early diagnosis and treatment of kidney disease can help to prevent serious complications.

Stages of kidney disease?

CKD(chronic kidney disease) is divided into five stages based on how well the kidneys are working. The stages are:

* **Stage 1:** Kidney damage with normal or increased GFR (>90 mL/min/1.73 m2)

* **Stage 2:** GFR is only slightly reduced (60–89 mL/min/1.73 m2)

* **Stage 3a:** Moderate reduction in GFR (45-59 mL/min/1.73 m2)

* **Stage 3b:** Moderate reduction in GFR (30-44 mL/min/1.73 m2)

* **Stage 4:** GFR severely reduced (15-29 mL/min/1.73 m2)

* **Stage 5:** Dialysis or kidney failure (GFR 15 mL/min/1.73 m2)

People with stage 1 CKD may not have any symptoms. As the disease progresses, people may experience symptoms such as fatigue, swelling, shortness of breath, and changes in urination.

There is no cure for CKD, but there are treatments that can help slow the progression of the disease and improve quality of life. CKD can be treated with medication, lifestyle modifications, dialysis, or kidney transplantation.

Consult your doctor if you have any worries regarding the condition of your kidneys.

Early diagnosis and treatment of CKD can help improve your chances of a good outcome.

Here are some additional information about each stage of CKD:

* **Stage 1:**

Kidney damage with normal or increased GFR (>90 mL/min/1.73 m2)

In stage 1 CKD, the kidneys are still working well enough to filter the blood effectively. However, there is some damage to the kidneys, which may be caused by high blood pressure, diabetes, or other diseases. People with stage 1 CKD may not have any symptoms.

* **Stage 2:**

GFR slightly decreased (60-89 mL/min/1.73 m2)

In stage 2 CKD, the kidneys are still working, but they are not working as well as they used to. The GFR is reduced, but it is still above 60 mL/min/1.73

m2. People with stage 2 CKD may not have any symptoms, or they may experience mild symptoms such as fatigue, swelling, and changes in urination.

* **Stage 3a:**

Moderate reduction in GFR (45-59 mL/min/1.73 m2)

In stage 3a CKD, the kidneys are working less well than they used to. The GFR is reduced to between 45 and 59 mL/min/1.73 m2. People with stage 3a CKD may experience more noticeable symptoms such as fatigue, swelling, shortness of breath, and changes in urination.

* **Stage 3b:**

Moderate reduction in GFR (30-44 mL/min/1.73 m2)

In stage 3b CKD, the kidneys are working even less well than they used to. The GFR is reduced to between 30 and 44 mL/min/1.73 m2. People with stage 3b CKD may experience more severe symptoms such as fatigue, swelling, shortness of breath, and changes in urination.

* Stage 4:

GFR severely reduced (15-29 mL/min/1.73 m2)

In stage 4 CKD, the kidneys are working very poorly. The GFR is reduced to between 15 and 29 mL/min/1.73 m2. People with stage 4 CKD may need to start dialysis or kidney transplant to survive.

* Stage 5:

Dialysis or kidney failure (GFR 15 mL/min/1.73 m2)

In stage 5 CKD, the kidneys have failed completely. GFR is less than 15 mL per minute per 1.73 m2. People with stage 5 CKD need to start dialysis or kidney transplant to survive.

Symptoms of kidney disease?

Here are a few signs of kidney disease:
- Fatigue
- Swelling in the feet, ankles, and hands

- Trouble sleeping
- Shortness of breath
- Loss of appetite
- Muscle cramps
- Dry, itchy skin
- Foamy urine
- Blood in the urine
- High blood pressure
- Frequent urination, especially at night
- Pain in the side or back
- Weight loss
- Confusion

Causes of kidney disease

Here are lists of the causes of kidney disease:
- Diabetes
- High blood pressure
- Heart disease
- Smoking
- Obesity

- Family history of kidney disease
- Abnormal kidney structure
- Older age
- Frequent use of medications that can damage the kidneys
- Infections
- Autoimmune diseases
- Genetic disorders
- Substance abuse
- Trauma
- Radiation exposure
- Toxins

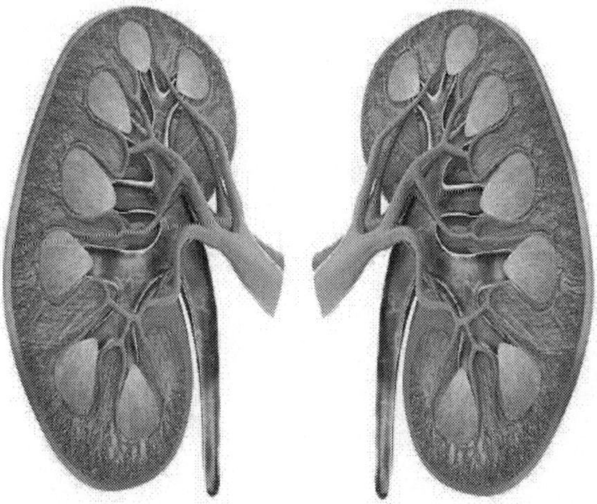

Treatment for kidney disease

Medications:

Medications can be used to control blood pressure, blood sugar, and cholesterol levels. These are important to control to slow the progression of kidney disease.

Diet:

A healthy diet can help to control blood pressure, blood sugar, and cholesterol levels. Additionally, it can aid in lowering the chance of acquiring kidney stones.

Exercise:

Exercise can help to control blood pressure, blood sugar, and cholesterol levels. Additionally, it can aid in lowering the chance of acquiring kidney stones.

Dialysis:

When the kidneys are unable to eliminate waste materials and excess fluid from the blood, a procedure called dialysis is used. Dialysis is classified into two types: hemodialysis and peritoneal dialysis.

Kidney transplant:

A kidney transplant is a surgical procedure that replaces a damaged kidney with a healthy kidney obtained from a donor. This is the most effective kidney failure treatment.

It is important to note that these are just some of the treatments for kidney disease. The best treatment for you will depend on the stage of your kidney disease and your individual needs.

Medications

Blood pressure medications:

These medications help to lower blood pressure, which can help to protect the kidneys from further damage. Some examples of blood pressure medications that are used to treat kidney disease include angiotensin-converting enzyme (ACE) inhibitors, angiotensin receptor blockers (ARBs), and calcium channel blockers.

Diabetes medications:
These medications help to control blood sugar levels, which can help to protect the kidneys from further damage. Some examples of diabetes medications that are used to treat kidney disease include insulin, metformin, and sulfonylurea drugs.

Statins:
These medications help to lower cholesterol levels, which can help to protect the kidneys from further damage. Some examples of statins that are used to

treat kidney disease include atorvastatin, simvastatin, and pravastatin.

Anaemia medications:
These medications help to produce more red blood cells, which can help to relieve fatigue and weakness associated with anaemia. Some examples of anaemia medications that are used to treat kidney disease include erythropoietin (EPO) and darbepoetin alfa.

Phosphorus binders:
These medications help to bind to phosphorus in the gut, which can help to lower phosphorus levels in the blood. Some examples of phosphorus binders that are used to treat kidney disease include calcium acetate, calcium carbonate, and sevelamer.

Vitamin D supplements:
These supplements help to keep bones healthy, which can help to reduce the risk of fractures. Some

examples of vitamin D supplements that are used to treat kidney disease include cholecalciferol (vitamin D3) and ergocalciferol (vitamin D2).

Diet

Here are some simple tips for a kidney-friendly diet:
- Eat plenty of fruits and vegetables.
- Select lean protein sources including fish, chicken, and legumes.
- Limit your consumption of processed meals, red meat, and sugary beverages.
- Drink plenty of water.
- Avoid foods heavy in salt, potassium, and phosphorus.

If you are concerned about your kidney health, consult your doctor or a certified dietician. They can help you create a personalised diet plan that meets your individual needs.

Here are some specific examples of foods that are good for your kidney:

Fruits: apples, bananas, berries, citrus fruits, grapes, melons, peaches, pears, plums, and tomatoes

Vegetables: leafy greens, broccoli, carrots, celery, cucumbers, eggplant, peppers, potatoes, squash, and sweet potatoes

Lean protein sources: fish, chicken, turkey, beans, lentils, and tofu

Low-fat dairy products: milk, yoghourt, and cheese

Whole grains: bread, pasta, rice, and cereal

Nuts and seeds

Healthy oils: olive oil, canola oil, and peanut oil

Foods to be avoided

Here are some examples of foods that you should limit or avoid if you have kidney problems:

Salty foods: processed foods, canned foods, and fast food

High-potassium foods: bananas, oranges, potatoes, tomatoes, and spinach

High-phosphorus foods: red meat, dairy products, and nuts

Sugary drinks: soda, juice, and sports drinks

Alcohol

Exercise

Exercise is an important part of kidney health. It can help to improve your blood pressure, control your blood sugar, and reduce your risk of heart disease. If you have kidney problems, exercise can help to slow the progression of the disease and improve your quality of life.

Here are some exercises that are good for your kidneys:

- Walking
- Swimming
- Biking
- Dancing
- Yoga
- Tai chi
- Pilates
- Strength training

These exercises are all low-impact and can be done at a variety of intensities. It is important to talk to your doctor before starting any new exercise program, especially if you have kidney problems.

Here are some additional tips for exercising with kidney problems:

- Begin slowly and progressively increase the intensity and duration of your workouts.
- Listen to your body and stop if you experience any pain.

- Stay hydrated by drinking plenty of water.
- Avoid exercising in hot weather.
- Talk to your doctor about any medications you are taking, as some of them can affect your ability to exercise.

Dialysis

Dialysis is a procedure that helps your body remove extra fluid and waste products from your blood when your kidneys are not able to. Dialysis can be done in a hospital, a dialysis centre, or at home. Based on your medical condition and preferences, you and your doctor will decide which type of dialysis and location is ideal for you.

There are two main types of dialysis: hemodialysis and peritoneal dialysis.

* **Hemodialysis** is a procedure that uses a machine to filter your blood. During hemodialysis, a needle is

inserted into your arm and a tube is attached to the needle. The tube is connected to a dialysis machine, which filters your blood and removes waste products and excess fluid. The filtered blood is then returned to your body through another tube. Hemodialysis treatments usually last for 3-4 hours and are typically done 3 times per week.

* **Peritoneal dialysis** is a procedure that uses your own body's tissues to filter your blood. During peritoneal dialysis, a catheter is inserted into your abdomen. The catheter is connected to a bag of dialysate solution, which is a fluid that contains sugar and other nutrients. The dialysate solution is then allowed to flow into your abdomen through the catheter. The waste products and excess fluid from your blood are then absorbed into the dialysate solution. After a few hours, the dialysate solution is drained back into the bag. Peritoneal dialysis can be

done at home and can be done continuously or intermittently.

Dialysis can have some side effects, including:
* Fatigue
* Muscle cramps
* Headaches
* Nausea
* Vomiting
* Dizziness
* Low blood pressure
* Infection
* Bleeding

Dialysis is a lifelong treatment for people with kidney failure. It is important to talk to your doctor about the risks and benefits of dialysis before deciding if it is right for you.

Kidney transplant

A kidney transplant is a procedure in which a diseased kidney is replaced with a healthy kidney from a living or deceased donor. It is a treatment option for people with end-stage renal disease (ESRD), which is a permanent condition in which the kidneys can no longer function properly.

<u>Living-donor transplants and deceased-donor transplants are the two forms of kidney transplants.</u>

Living-donor transplants are when a healthy person donates one of their kidneys to a loved one or friend. Deceased-donor transplants are when a kidney is donated from someone who has died.

The kidney transplant surgery is typically performed laparoscopically, which means that it is done through small incisions in the abdomen. The donor kidney is placed in the lower abdomen and the blood vessels and ureter are connected to the recipient's blood vessels and bladder.

Kidney transplants are generally very successful. The success rate for living-donor transplants is about 95% at five years, and the success rate for deceased-donor transplants is about 85% at five years.

<u>Kidney transplants can offer many benefits to patients, including:</u>
- Improved quality of life
- Increased life expectancy
- Reduced need for dialysis
- Reduced risk of death

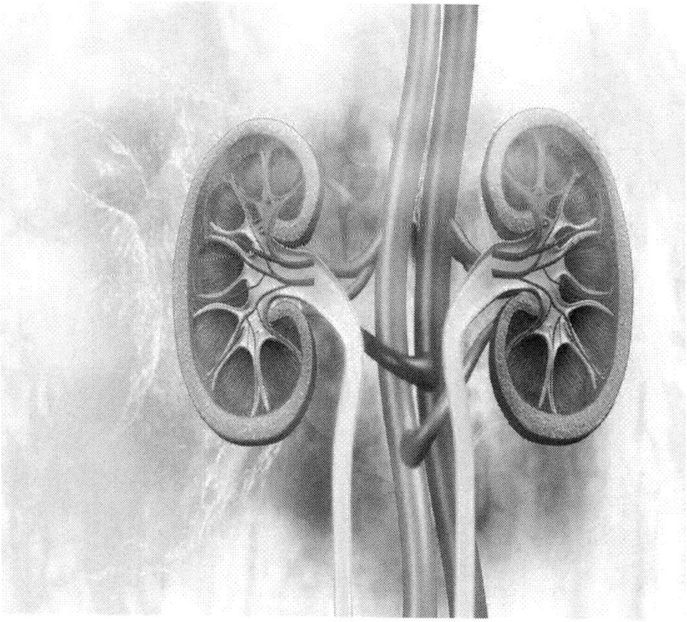

Prevention Of Kidney Disease

- Control your blood pressure
- Control your blood sugar
- Eat a healthy diet
- Exercise regularly
- Don't smoke
- Lose weight if you are overweight or obese
- Get regular checkups

Control your blood pressure. High blood pressure can damage your kidneys over time.

Control your blood sugar. Diabetes can damage your kidneys.

Quit smoking. Smoking can damage your kidneys.

Eat a healthy diet. A healthy diet can help keep your blood pressure and blood sugar under control.

Get regular exercise. Exercise can help keep your blood pressure and blood sugar under control.

Lose weight if you are overweight or obese. Excess weight can put extra strain on your kidneys.

Avoid taking over-the-counter pain relievers without talking to your doctor. Some over-the-counter pain relievers, such as ibuprofen and naproxen, can damage your kidneys if taken in high doses or for long periods of time.

Get regular checkups. Your doctor can check your kidney function and make sure you are doing everything you can to prevent kidney disease.

Conclusion

Kidney disease is a serious condition, but it can be managed with proper treatment and care.

If you have kidney disease, it is important to work with your doctor to create a treatment plan that is right for you.

With proper care, you can live a long and healthy life with kidney disease.

The future of kidney disease

The future of kidney disease is promising. There are many new technologies and treatments being developed that have the potential to improve the lives of people with kidney disease.

Some of the most promising developments include:

Artificial kidneys:

Artificial kidneys are machines that can mimic the function of the human kidney. They are currently in the early stages of development, but they have the potential to revolutionise the treatment of kidney disease.

Gene therapy:

Gene therapy is a treatment that uses genetic engineering to correct or replace defective genes. It is being investigated as a potential treatment for a variety of kidney diseases, including polycystic kidney disease and Alport syndrome.

Regenerative medicine:

Regenerative medicine is a branch of medicine concerned with the repair or replacement of damaged tissues and organs. It is being investigated as a potential treatment for kidney disease, and there have been some promising results in early clinical trials.

These are just a few of the many new developments that are being made in the field of kidney disease. With continued research and development, it is likely that the future of kidney disease will be bright.

<u>In addition to these new technologies, there are also a number of other things that can be done to improve the future of kidney disease. These include:</u>

Early detection:
Early detection of kidney disease is essential for improving outcomes. People with early-stage kidney disease often have no symptoms, so it is important to get regular checkups and blood tests.

Prevention:

There are a number of things that can be done to prevent kidney disease, including:

- Controlling blood pressure
- Managing diabetes
- Avoiding smoking
- Eating a healthy diet
- Exercising regularly

By taking these steps, we can help to prevent kidney disease and improve the future of kidney disease for everyone.

Hope and healing for people with kidney disease

There is hope and healing for people with kidney disease. With early detection and treatment, many people with kidney disease can live long and healthy lives. There are also a number of new treatments being developed that have the potential to improve the lives of people with kidney disease.

Here are some things that people with kidney disease can do to improve their health and well-being:

Get regular checkups and blood tests.

This is important for early detection of kidney disease and to monitor the progression of the disease.

Take medications as prescribed.

This is important for controlling blood pressure, blood sugar, and other risk factors for kidney disease.

Eat a healthy diet.

This involves consuming an abundance of fruits, vegetables, and whole grains. It is also important to limit processed foods, sugary drinks, and salt.

Exercise regularly.

Exercise helps to control blood pressure, blood sugar, and cholesterol. It also contributes to better overall health and well-being.

Quit smoking.

Smoking damages the kidneys and increases the risk of kidney disease.

Manage stress.

Stress can worsen kidney disease. There are a number of ways to manage stress, such as exercise, relaxation techniques, and spending time with loved ones.

There are also a number of support groups available for people with kidney disease. These groups can provide emotional support, information, and resources.

If you or someone you know has kidney disease, there is hope and healing. With early detection and treatment, many people with kidney disease can live long and healthy lives.

STAY SAFE!!

NOTE

NOTE

NOTE

Made in United States
Orlando, FL
29 May 2025